COVID-19 VS MONKEYPOX VIRUS: Key Differences Between the Trending Pandemics

DORA SMITH

All rights reserved. No part of this publication may be reproduced, distributed, or transmitted in any form or by any means, including photocopying, recording, or other electronic or mechanical methods, without the prior written permission of the publisher, except in the case of brief quotations embodied in critical reviews and certain other noncommercial uses permitted by copyright law.

Copyright © Dora Smith, 2022.

TABLE OF CONTENT

ABSTRACT

CHAPTER ONE : ALL YOU NEED TO KNOW ABOUT THE PANDEMICS

CHAPTER TWO: KEY DIFFERENCES BETWEEN THE PANDEMICS

REFERENCE

ABSTRACT

The continuous outbreaks of zoonotic infectious disease pose a huge public health risk. several viral sicknesses with epidemic potential are undermining worldwide health security. Zoonotic viruses, specifically, have caused various epidemics in the present years, bringing about high morbidity and mortality. The COVID-19 pandemic demonstrated that any infection outbreak that can transmit human-to-human or with cross-species transmission capacity could cause critical risks and add to a global pandemic.

A few nations have not completely recovered from the COVID-19 emergency yet. The COVID-19 pandemic has brought about enormous misfortunes with regards to human life and economy in United States. In spite of the fact that lessons are being learnt from every infection episode, the repetitive outbreak of new or reemerging viruses act as a wakeup call that zoonotic pathogens will keep on emerging. Two long years after sustaining through the COVID-19 pandemic, another zoonotic monkeypox virus transmission has been reported in numerous non-endemic countries lately. In spite of the fact that it is an uncommon, self-restricting disease, normally milder than smallpox and not a worry at this stage, early detection and quick response is critical for the virus control.

My book is focused on the discoveries, risks and the key differences between COVID -19 and monkeypox virus.I briefly enlightened my reader's on the preventive measures to apply for a better health security.

CHAPTER ONE

INTRODUCTION

ALL YOU NEED TO KNOW ABOUT THE PANDEMICS

The COVID-19 epidemic started at Wuhan, China and within a few months became a worldwide pandemic. The World Health Organization (WHO) proclaim the COVID-19 outbreak as a public health hazard of international concern on the 30th of January, 2020. At this time, 34 regions in China had reported infections and the total number of cases surpasses that for the 2003 Severe Acute Respiratory Syndrome (SARS). On the same day, United States Centers for Disease Control and Prevention (CDC) confirmed the first case of human to human transmission in United States. On the 31th of January, 2020 Health and

Human Services (HHS) declared Coronavirus a global health emergency in United States. Also, on the same day, CDC issued a federal quarantine for 2 weeks affecting 195 American evacuees from Wuhan, China. The first COVID-19 death in United States of America was reported on the 29th of February, 2020. Over the next 71 days, the virus hit United States of America especially hard resulting in 80,787 deaths and over 1.36 million infections. During pandemics it is usual for healthcare providers and scientists to primarily focus on the pathogen to study its mechanism with an aim of containing it and treating the disease.

An unusual and life-threatening viral disease, monkeypox has been recently discovered in more than 12 non-African countries. Monkeypox is a communicable disease caused by the monkeypox virus. There is recently an outbreak of monkeypox in the U.S. and other nation where the virus is not usually seen. Fever, headache, muscle aches and backache, swollen lymph nodes, chills, exhaustion, a rash that can look like pimples or blisters that appears on the face, inside the mouth, and on other parts of the body, like the hands, feet, chest, genitals, or anus are the symptoms of monkeypox.

WHO has confirmed more than 123 cases of monkeypox (both suspected or confirmed cases) from countries viz., Australia, Belgium, Canada, France, Germany, Italy, Netherland, Portugal, Spain, Sweden, the UK, and the USA. The highest number of cases has been reported from Portugal, Spain, and recently, a report informed that it might be a community transmission in the UK. Nevertheless, from the literature search, it was found that most cases of human monkeypox, which have been reported from time to time, are observed in West Africa and Central Africa that are endemic regions for this virus.

This zoonotic virus was first discovered in 1958 in the monkey colonies, which were preserved in a Danish research laboratory, and pox-like disease was observed. Therefore, the condition was named as 'Monkeypox.' However, this discovery of monkeypox case was from an animal. The first human case was reported when the virus was identified in a child from Congo (DRC) in 1970. Monkeypox virus belongs to the genus *Orthopoxvirus* and is a member of the family Poxviridae. Two clades are noted in this virus: the first is the Congo Basin clade (also entitled as Central African clade), and the other is the West African clade. The virus has double-stranded DNA (dsDNA), and the sequence of the genome length is about 1,97,124 bp.

Some researchers have reported that air travel is the source of the spread of infectious diseases. Recently, due to the increase of the global population, the networks for transportation have increased. Air travel has played a notable role among transportation networks. Due to the increasing affordability and effortlessness, air travel has created faster and easier mobility for people. Owing to air travel and mobility of people, different zoonotic infectious diseases, vector-borne, food-borne, and air-borne diseases have been reported to be transmitted during air travel. However, the medical community and aviation industry should train or enlighten the ordinary individuals regarding health issues related to air travel. They should be educated on how to prevent and control the air travel related infections.

CHAPTER TWO

KEY DIFFERENCES BETWEEN THE PANDEMICS

The sudden emergence of monkeypox can be alarming after over two years of living through the COVID-19 pandemic, monkeypox is not a new virus and does not spread in the same way as COVID-19. The table below shows the key differences between monkeypox virus and COVID-19.

S/N	FACTORS	MONKEYPOX VIRUS	COVID-19
1	**Widespread rate**	Typically found in central and western African countries. From May 2022, new cases have been identified in many other countries, including the U.S. However, monkeypox is	More than hundred million cases have been recorded since the start of the pandemic and still spreading widely throughout the world.

		much less common than COVID-19.	
2	**Year of Identification**	Since 1958	Since 2019
3	**Mode of transmission**	1) Close physical/intimate contacts e.g. skin-to-skin contact including sex 2) Contact with contaminated	Extremely infectious. Can spread from people with the virus, even if they don't have symptoms through tiny droplets in

		materials (towels, bedding and clothing) 3) Respiratory droplets spread by close and prolonged face-to-face contact	the air by breathing, talking, sneezing, or coughing.
4	**Signs and symptoms**	1) Rashes and lesions with firm bumps on face, hands,	1) Fever 2) Cough

		feet, skin, or genitals	3) Breathing difficulties
		2) Fever	4) Stomach issues
		3) Swollen lymph nodes	5) Headaches
		4) Chills	6) Muscle aches
		5) Low energy	7) Loss of taste and smell
			8) Cold symptoms

| 5. | Variants | All viruses change and evolve over time. The monkeypox virus mutates slower than coronaviruses. There are two known "clades" of monkeypox virus. The clade recently identified in Europe, Canada, and in the United | There are many variants of SARS-CoV-2. This virus mutates rapidly. |

		States is the West African clade, which tends to cause less severe disease.	
6	**Preventive Measures**	Avoid close physical contact with people who have symptoms, includin	Get tested, vaccinated and boosted

		g sores or rashes	Always wear a mask at indoor settings and crowded outdoor settings
		Ensure that you update your sexual partner/s about any recent illness and be careful of new or	

		sudden sores or rashes Avoid getting in contact with contaminated materials Always wear mask,	☐ Always meet people outdoors or in well ventilated spaces

		gloves etc. if you can't avoid close contact with someone who has symptoms ☐ Always practice good	

	hand hygiene	

CONCLUSION

Before long, we will acquire lucidity on the magnitude of the ongoing outbreak as case tracking down escalates. Acting rapidly and proactively will be urgent for containing it. Guaranteeing that we learn from ongoing pandemics and their differences. Also sharing accessible resources early and immediately will be a better way to progress. The admonition signals on monkeypox turning into a worldwide general health concern have been available for many years.

Right now, is an ideal opportunity to embrace a really worldwide methodology that resolves this issue conclusively in wealthy nations as well as, basically, in the endemic nations that have been responding to monkeypox and covid-19 for quite a long time.

REFERENCE

Manojit Bhattacharya, Kuldeep Dhama, and Chiranjib Chakraborty (2022). *Recently spreading human monkeypox virus infection and its transmission during COVID-19 pandemic period: A travelers' prospective. Journal of Travel Med Infect Dis.* Pp.18-38 https://doi.org/10.1016/j.tmaid.2022.102398

Wagner Gouvea dos Santos (2020) *Natural history of COVID-19 and current knowledge on treatment therapeutic options. Journal of Biomedicine & Pharmacotherapy* pp 62-197.https://www.doi:10.1016/j.biopha.2020.110493

World Health Organization (2022). *Disease Outbreak News; Multi-country monkeypox outbreak in non-endemic countries*: Update. Available at https://www.who.int/emergencies/disease-outbreak-news/item/2022-DON393

Boghuma K Titanji, Bryan Tegomoh, Saman Nematollahi, Michael Konomos, Prathit A

Kulkarni (2022). *Monkeypox: A Contemporary Review for Healthcare Professionals. Journal of open forum infectious diseases.* vol 9(7) https://doi.org/10.1093/ofid/ofac310

University Hospitals (2022). *Monkeypox and COVID-19: Here Are Key Differences. Journal of science of health, the Art of compassion.*

Shanmugaraj B, Khorattanakulchai N, Phoolcharoen W. (2022). *Emergence of monkeypox: Another concern amidst COVID-19 crisis. Asian Pac J Trop Med* [serial online].5(15) https://www.apjtm.org/text.asp?2022/15/5/193/346081

Barnali Bhattacharjee , Tathagata Acharya (2020) .*The COVID-19 Pandemic and its Effect on Mental Health in USA – A Review with Some Coping Strategies. Journal of Psychiatric Quarterly.* Vol 91 pp 1135-1145. https://doi.org/10.1007/s11126-020-09836-0

www.ingramcontent.com/pod-product-compliance
Lightning Source LLC
Chambersburg PA
CBHW050328220526
45465CB00005B/2181